KNOWLEDGE GUIDE TO HERNIATED DISC

Essential Manual To Pain Relief, Treatment Options, Exercises, And Long Term Recovery Strategies

DR. AARON BRANUM

Copyright © 2024 BY DR. AARON BRANUM

All rights reserved. Except for brief quotations embodied in critical reviews and certain other noncommercial uses permitted by copyright law, no part of this publication may be reproduced, distributed, or transmitted in any form or by any means, Including photocopying, recording, or other electronic or mechanical methods, without the prior written permission of the publisher.

Disclaimer:

The data in this book, is solely meant to be informative and instructional.

This book is not intended to replace expert medical advice, diagnosis, or care. No medical, health, or other professional services are offered by the author, publisher, or any affiliated parties

Individual outcomes may differ in the practice of these therapies, which entail a variety of approaches and methodologies.

A one-on-one session with a trained or certified healthcare professional is still preferable. It is best to consult a trained healthcare provider before making any decisions regarding your health.

The author of this book is not affiliated with any specific website, product, or organization related to any of these therapies.

All reasonable measures have been taken by the author and publisher to guarantee the authenticity and dependability of the material contained in this book

Contents

CHAPTER ONE 13
THE SPINE'S ANATOMY 13
- An Overview Of The Spinal Structure 14
- Intervertebral Disc Functions 15
- Comprehending Disc Degeneration 16
- Nerves' Function In Spinal Health 17

CHAPTER TWO 19
INDICATES AND SYMPTOMS 19
- Typical Herniated Disc Symptoms............ 20
- Distinguishing Herniated Disc From Other Spinal Disorders 21
- Recognizing Warning Signs..................... 22
- Effects On Activities Of Daily Life............. 23
- When To Get Medical Help...................... 24

CHAPTER THREE 27
DIAGNOSTIC METHODS 27
- Methods Of Physical Examination 30
- Imaging Investigations: CT, MRI, And X-Rays 33

   Nerve Conduction Studies (NCS) And
   Electromyography (EMG) 35

   The Myelography And Discography 38

CHAPTER FOUR 43

  CAREFUL MANAGEMENT 43

   Pain Relief Techniques: Pharmaceuticals And
   Physiotherapy 43

   Lifestyle Changes: Exercise, Weight
   Management, And Posture 45

   Acupuncture And Chiropractic Care 47

   Steroid Injections Epidural 48

CHAPTER FIVE 51

  SURGICAL MEDICATION ACTIONS 51

   Surgical Procedure Types 51

   Benefits And Risks Of Surgery 52

   Surgery Preparation: What To Expect 53

   Rehabilitation And Postoperative Care 54

   Other Surgical Choices 55

CHAPTER SIX 57

  REPAY AND RESUMMATION 57

Early Stage Recuperation: Rest And Adjustment Of Activities 57

Exercises In Physical Therapy For Strengthening And Flexibility 58

Pain Control Throughout Healing 59

Resuming Regular Activities: Employment, Athletics, And Leisure 60

Extended-Duration Rehabilitative Techniques 61

CHAPTER SEVEN 65

PREVENTIVE ACTIONS 65

The Value Of Preserving Spinal Health 66

Ergonomic Advice For Preventing Injuries . 67

Stretching And Exercise Programmes 68

Supplements And Diet For Healthy Spine .. 69

Frequent Inspections And Surveillance 70

CHAPTER EIGHT 73

MANAGING METHODS AND ASSISTANCE 73

Coping Strategies And Psychological Effects Of Chronic Pain 75

Peer Networks And Support Groups 76

Interacting With Healthcare Professionals . 77

Maintaining A Healthy Emotional And
Physical State 79

Integrating Self-Care Into Daily Routine ... 80

CHAPTER NINE 83

COMMONLY ASKED QUESTIONS OR FAQS .. 83

Can A Disc Herniation Heal By Itself? 83

How Much Time Does It Take To Recover
From Surgery? 84

Exist Any Activities I Should Stay Away
From? 85

Is It Possible To Stop Herniated Discs From
Recurring? 86

If Conservative Treatments Don't Work,
What Should I Do? 87

In the enormous sea of spinal health, the "Knowledge Guide to Herniated Disc" is a beacon of insight. Its main focus is on providing a thorough understanding of the complexities surrounding herniated discs, including their nature, causes, symptoms, and diagnosis. Through exploring these domains, readers acquire a deep understanding of what a herniated disc actually is and how it affects their lives.

Navigating the field of spinal health requires an understanding of the anatomy of the spine. With a perceptive synopsis of the anatomy of the spine and an explanation of the vital function of intervertebral discs, readers are taken on a deep dive into the complexities of the spinal system. This chapter explains how discs degenerate and the complex interaction between spinal nerves that leads to herniated discs.

Symptoms and indicators act as early warning signs of spinal distress, directing people to seek treatment as soon as possible. This book equips readers with the information to recognize warning signs and take preventative action by outlining typical symptoms and clarifying the subtle differences in distinguishing from other spine disorders. Additionally, it highlights how herniated discs affect activities of daily living and stresses the significance of early intervention.

In the maze of spinal health, diagnostic methods serve as the compass, pointing medical professionals in the direction of precise evaluations and individualized treatment regimens. Through elucidating the complexities of physical examination methods and imaging tests like CT, MRI, and X-rays, readers are able to comprehend the diagnosis process. It emphasizes how crucial it is to understand test results, which highlights how crucial it is to make well-informed decisions.

Conservative treatments emerge as reliable friends in the fight against herniated discs with the goal of holistic care. People get relief by using a multimodal strategy that includes lifestyle changes, chiropractic adjustments, and acupuncture in addition to traditional pain management techniques. To promote a balanced viewpoint, the guide clearly outlines the advantages and restrictions of conservative therapy.

Those suffering from severe disc herniation have hope thanks to surgical procedures.

People are better able to navigate the surgical landscape when the different types of surgical treatments, together with their associated risks, advantages, and alternatives, are explained. Furthermore, knowledge of preoperative planning and postoperative care promotes a smooth transition from illness to rehabilitation.

The key to living a life free from spinal problems is recovery and rehabilitation. Through an investigation into physical therapy exercises, long-term rehabilitation tactics, and early-stage recovery, people set out on a revolutionary path toward enhanced functionality. The guide also emphasizes the value of prevention, giving readers the tools they need to protect their spinal health with regular check-ups, exercise regimens, and ergonomic practices.

Support and coping mechanisms act as life preservers, pointing people towards safety amongst harsh waters of long-term discomfort and psychological turmoil. Through clarifying coping strategies, resources for assistance, and the practice of self-care, the manual equips readers to weather adversity with fortitude and poise.

FAQs give people a way to find their way around the world of herniated discs by answering their most common questions about everything from post-surgical recovery to natural healing processes. The book gives those who are just starting out on their path to spinal wellness confidence by providing accurate and compassionate answers to frequently asked questions.

CHAPTER ONE
THE SPINE'S ANATOMY

Knowing the structure of the spine is essential to understanding the effects of herniated discs on the body. With its 33 vertebrae stacked on top of one another, the spine is an amazing structure. The five areas of these vertebrae are: sacral, lumbar (lower back), thoracic (upper back), cervical (neck), and coccygeal (tailbone).

The spinal cord travels through the hollow center of each vertebra, which is shielded by a network of bony rings known as the vertebral arches. The spinal canal, which is formed by these arches, protects the spinal cord from harm. An intervertebral disc sits in between each pair of vertebrae, allowing the spine to be stable, and flexible, and function as shock absorbers.

An Overview Of The Spinal Structure

Because of its construction, the spine can be compared to a column that supports the body and permits movement in all directions while being stable. Most of the weight of the body is supported by the vertebral bodies, which are the biggest portion of each vertebra. In the meantime, forces are distributed and the appropriate distance between vertebrae is maintained by the intervertebral discs, which are located in between them.

The spinal cord, a crucial component of the central nervous system that carries out signal transmission from the brain to the body's other organs, is also housed in the spinal column.

The meninges and cerebrospinal fluid, two layers of tissue that surround the spinal cord, act as additional cushions and supports.

Intervertebral Disc Functions

Intervertebral discs are essential for the health of the spine in multiple ways. They serve as shock absorbers, protecting the spine from blows and averting injury when in motion. These discs also provide flexibility, which makes it possible for the spine to effortlessly twist, bend, and rotate.

The nucleus pulposus, a gel-like substance, is enclosed by a stiff outer layer termed the annulus fibrosus, which makes up the construction of intervertebral discs.

The discs' exceptional composition allows them to resist compressive forces without losing their integrity or shape.

Comprehending Disc Degeneration

In addition to being a normal aspect of aging, disc degeneration can also be brought on by trauma or prolonged pressure.

Our intervertebral discs lose elasticity and durability as we age because their water content drops. This degradation can result in a lower disc height, less capacity to absorb trauma, and a higher risk of herniation.

The rate of disc degeneration can be influenced by a variety of factors, including work, lifestyle decisions, and heredity.

It is well recognized that smoking, obesity, and bad posture hasten this process; nevertheless, regular exercise and ergonomic practices can help lessen its consequences.

Nerves' Function In Spinal Health

Since nerves carry motor signals and sensory data from the brain to the rest of the body, they are essential to spinal health. The spinal cord is a collection of nerves that are housed in the spinal canal and shielded from harm by the soft tissues and surrounding bones.

At different levels, peripheral nerves emerge from the spinal cord and go to distinct parts of the body. These neurons regulate muscle function and movement in addition to transmitting sensations including pain, touch, and temperature.

The Causes of Herniated Discs

Herniated discs happen when an intervertebral disc's soft inner core pushes through a rip or weak spot in the outer covering. This protrusion may compress adjacent spinal nerves, resulting in pain, tingling, weakness, or numbness in the affected area.

A herniated disc can occur as a result of a number of circumstances, such as age-related degeneration, acute injury, incorrect lifting technique, and repetitive stress. Due to the excessive strain they place on the spine, poor posture and sedentary lifestyle choices can further raise the risk of disc herniation.

Effective management of herniated discs requires an early diagnosis and proper therapy. To reduce symptoms and encourage healing, conservative methods like rest, physical therapy, and medication are frequently enough. In more extreme situations, spinal nerve pressure may need to be relieved surgically in order to regain function.

CHAPTER TWO
INDICATES AND SYMPTOMS

Depending on the location and severity of the disc herniation, a herniated disc may present with a number of signs and symptoms. Pain, which can be localized or radiated throughout the afflicted nerve pathway, is one of the most prevalent complaints. This discomfort, which is frequently made worse by particular motions or postures, can range from mild and achy to severe and shooting.

Numbness or tingling, usually seen in the extremities that correspond to the damaged nerve roots, is another characteristic symptom. For example, a herniation in the cervical spine may result in comparable symptoms in the arms or hands, whereas one in the lumbar spine may induce tingling or numbness in the legs. In addition to these sensory abnormalities, people may also feel weakness in their muscles, especially in the regions that are supplied by the damaged nerves.

Typical Herniated Disc Symptoms

Herniated discs most frequently cause localized or radiating pain, which is frequently characterized as a sharp or burning feeling. Certain activities, such as lifting, bending, or extended sitting or standing, can make this pain worse. Muscle spasms in the afflicted area are another common complaint, which can worsen pain and reduce range of motion.

Herniated discs typically result in tingling or numbness along the afflicted nerve's path in addition to pain. Depending on where the herniation is, this feeling, called radiculopathy, may radiate from the spine into the arms or legs. In addition to these sensory abnormalities, the affected area may have muscle weakness that makes it challenging to carry out daily chores or engage in physical activity.

Distinguishing Herniated Disc From Other Spinal Disorders

Herniated discs can be diagnosed with the use of specific distinguishing characteristics, even though they share some symptoms with other spinal disorders. For instance, radicular pain—pain that travels along a particular nerve pathway—is frequently used as a diagnostic tool for disc herniation. Depending on where the herniation is, this pain might have a regular pattern that helps identify it from more widespread back discomfort.

Imaging tests, such as CT or MRI scans, can also give important information about the differences between other spinal diseases and herniated discs. These examinations can show the intervertebral discs' structure and detect any anomalies, such as protrusions or bulging, that may be signs of herniation. Furthermore, neurological exams can assist in determining the underlying source of symptoms by evaluating sensation, muscular strength, and reflexes.

Recognizing Warning Signs

Even though herniated discs are common and frequently go away with conservative therapy, there are some warning signs that could point to a more serious underlying issue that has to be treated right away. Progressive weakness or numbness is one of these warning signs; it should be taken especially seriously if it affects both sides of the body or is accompanied by bladder or bowel issues.

Loss of control over one's bowel or bladder is another worrisome symptom that could be cauda equina syndrome, an uncommon but dangerous consequence of severe disc herniation. Furthermore, an immediate evaluation is necessary to rule out fractures or other spinal cord damage in cases of abrupt onset of acute back pain, particularly following trauma or injury.

Effects On Activities Of Daily Life

Herniated discs can seriously impair day-to-day activities, including productivity at work and enjoyment of recreational activities. Simple activities like lifting, bending, and prolonged sitting can become difficult and uncomfortable for a lot of people. Productivity may decrease as a result, and living quality may deteriorate.

Herniated disc restrictions can also make it difficult to engage in hobbies and other pastimes, which can cause dissatisfaction and a sense of loss. Sports and gardening are two examples of activities that may need to be adjusted or avoided completely in order to prevent more pain and damage.

When To Get Medical Help

For a herniated disc to be diagnosed and treated quickly, it is imperative to know when to seek medical help. Seeking medical attention is crucial if symptoms worsen over time or if they don't go away with conservative treatments like rest, ice, and over-the-counter pain relievers.

In order to rule out more serious consequences, any red signs, such as growing weakness, numbness, or loss of control over one's bowels or bladder, should also prompt an immediate medical evaluation.

It is imperative to get medical attention as soon as possible if there are concerns about a herniated disc because prompt action can help prevent long-term harm and improve results.

CHAPTER THREE
DIAGNOSTIC METHODS

In order to effectively diagnose a herniated disc, medical professionals utilize a number of procedures. Thorough physical examinations are one of the main approaches. This entails evaluating your reflexes, muscular strength, range of motion, and sensation in the afflicted location. Physicians can frequently obtain important information regarding the existence and location of a herniated disc by closely analyzing these features.

Imaging studies are essential for diagnosis in addition to physical examination. An X-ray can show any anomalies, such as bone spurs or spinal canal narrowing, and can also give a general review of the structure of the spine. However, computed tomography (CT) and magnetic resonance imaging (MRI) are usually used to get a more detailed view of soft tissues like discs. With the use of these sophisticated imaging methods, medical practitioners can clearly see the spinal discs and determine the extent of herniations.

To assess nerve function and identify any anomalies, nerve conduction studies (NCS) and electromyography (EMG) are occasionally performed. These tests assist physicians in determining whether and to what degree nerve compression caused by a herniated disc is present. They do this by monitoring the electrical activity of muscles and the speed at which nerves communicate messages.

Discography and myelography can be used when conventional imaging examinations are not definitive or when more information is required. In myelography, dye is injected into the spinal canal to view the spinal cord and nerve roots; in discography, a contrast dye is injected into the damaged disc or discs to highlight any tears or leaks.

The specific location and severity of a disc herniation can be precisely determined with the help of these methods.

It's crucial to appropriately interpret the test results after it's all over. The presence, location, and severity of a herniated disc are identified by healthcare professionals after carefully examining the results.

Comprehending these findings is essential to creating a successful treatment strategy catered to the specific requirements of each patient.

Methods Of Physical Examination

A physical examination is essential to the diagnosis of a herniated disc because it gives medical professionals important information about a patient's symptoms and enables them to identify the underlying source of pain. Many methods are used to evaluate the spine's range of motion, muscular strength, reflexes, and feeling during a physical examination.

Evaluating the patient's range of motion is one of the main goals of a physical examination for a suspected herniated disc.

This entails asking the patient to carry out particular motions, including bending to the sides, backward, and forward, in order to assess any pain or limits related to these movements. A herniated disc may be present if there is a limited range of motion or if particular actions cause the symptoms to worsen.

Testing for muscle strength is yet another crucial component of the physical examination. To measure the strength of certain muscle groups in the affected area, medical professionals often ask patients to undertake a variety of strength exercises, such as pushing against resistance or lifting their legs. A herniated disc may be the cause of weakness or loss of strength in specific muscles, which may indicate nerve compression.

Additionally frequently carried out during a physical examination is reflex testing. Reflex hammers are used by medical professionals to trigger reflex responses in particular regions, such as the knees and ankles. Reflex alterations, such as lessened or heightened reflexes, may be a sign of nerve involvement linked to a herniated disc.

To assess the patient's sensation in the impacted area, sensory testing is done. In order to evaluate the patient's capacity to perceive touch, pressure, and pain in various body parts, medical professionals may employ a gentle brush or a pinprick.

Changes in feeling, including tingling or numbness, maybe a sign of a herniated disc compressing the nerves.

In general, a comprehensive physical examination helps medical professionals diagnose and treat a herniated disc by providing important details regarding a patient's symptoms, functional limits, and neurological state.

Imaging Investigations: CT, MRI, And X-Rays

Because imaging investigations provide precise visualizations of the spine and adjacent tissues, they are essential in the diagnosis of a herniated disc. X-rays, computed tomography (CT) scans, and magnetic resonance imaging (MRI) are the three main imaging modalities employed in this situation.

X-rays are frequently the initial imaging test carried out to evaluate the spine's general structure. Although X-rays cannot directly see soft tissues like discs, they can show any anomalies in the skeleton or misalignments that may be causing discomfort. For instance, X-rays can identify fractures, bone spurs, or spinal canal constrictions that could be a sign of a herniated disc.

The best imaging technique for assessing soft tissues, such as spinal discs, is magnetic resonance imaging (MRI). Healthcare professionals can see bulges, herniations, and other anomalies thanks to the thorough images it offers of the spinal cord, nerve roots, and intervertebral discs. When evaluating the degree of nerve compression and the severity of a herniated disc, magnetic resonance imaging (MRI) is especially helpful.

When further information is required or an MRI is not recommended, CT scans can also be used to diagnose a herniated disc. CT scans give precise cross-sectional pictures of the spine, which are useful for determining the degree of disc herniation and other bone structures. Myelography, which involves injecting a contrast dye into the spinal canal to improve the visibility of the spinal cord and nerve roots, may occasionally be used in conjunction with CT scans.

Every imaging modality has benefits and drawbacks, and the selection of an imaging study is influenced by a number of variables, such as the patient's symptoms, medical background, and requirement for comprehensive anatomical data. Healthcare professionals are able to effectively identify a herniated disc and provide a personalized treatment strategy for each patient by closely examining the images from X-rays, MRIs, or CT scans.

Nerve Conduction Studies (NCS) And Electromyography (EMG)

To evaluate nerve function and identify anomalies linked to a herniated disc, diagnostic techniques such as nerve conduction studies

(NCS) and electromyography (EMG) are invaluable. These examinations offer precise measurements of muscle and nerve activity, assisting medical professionals in identifying and assessing the extent of nerve compression.

In order to assess the electrical activity of certain muscles both at rest and during contraction, tiny needle electrodes are inserted into the muscles. A herniated disc can cause nerve irritation or injury, and EMG can detect these locations by analyzing the pattern and amplitude of muscle responses. Atypical EMG observations, including erratic activity or a decrease in muscle fiber recruitment, could point to nerve compression or malfunction.

In contrast, NCS measures the strength and speed of nerve impulses as they pass via nerve channels. Little electrical shocks are applied to the skin covering the nerves using electrodes during NCS in order to evaluate the reaction of the nerve. Healthcare professionals can detect areas of nerve compression or damage linked to a herniated disc by measuring the speed and amplitude of nerve transmission.

In order to provide a thorough assessment of nerve function and the location of nerve compression, EMG and NCS are frequently conducted in tandem.

These tests can support the diagnosis of a herniated disc, help distinguish it from other disorders that present with similar symptoms and assist in determining the best course of therapy. Furthermore, EMG and NCS can be useful instruments for tracking nerve regeneration and evaluating the effectiveness of treatments over time.

Despite the fact that EMG and NCS are usually safe and well-tolerated, some patients may feel some slight discomfort or short-term tightness in their muscles during the process. Nonetheless, the advantages of acquiring precise diagnostic data surpass the possible hazards, enabling medical professionals to create customized therapy strategies meant to alleviate symptoms and enhance functional results for individuals suffering from a herniated disc.

The Myelography And Discography

Specialized imaging techniques called discography and myelography are employed to assess spinal discs and associated structures when results from conventional imaging investigations are unclear or require more information. These diagnostic tests are very helpful in determining the exact location and degree of disc herniation, which helps with the diagnosis and treatment of disorders like herniated discs.

Under fluoroscopic supervision, a contrast dye is injected into the damaged disc or discs during a discography procedure. The dye fills the disc space, bringing attention to any holes, leaks, or structural irregularities in the disc. Healthcare professionals can determine the precise position and degree of disc herniation, as well as evaluate the integrity and function of the disc, by observing these alterations on imaging.

In contrast, a contrast dye is injected into the spinal canal around the spinal cord and nerve roots during a myelography procedure. During imaging investigations, this dye highlights the spinal cord and nerve roots, making any compression or displacement brought on by a herniated disc or other spinal abnormalities clearly visible. Computed tomography (CT) scans and myelography are frequently combined to improve image quality and provide more anatomical detail.

Discography and myelography are invasive procedures that entail some hazards, including the possibility of an injection site infection or allergic responses to the contrast dye.

These dangers are, nevertheless, rather minimal, and getting correct diagnostic information can frequently be more beneficial than harmful, particularly when conventional imaging studies haven't been able to provide enough clarity.

Diskography and myelography results must be interpreted with specific knowledge and training.

In order to identify the existence, location, and degree of a disc herniation as well as any related compression of the spinal cord or nerve roots, healthcare professionals carefully review the imaging results.

Having this information is essential for creating a personalized treatment plan that maximizes results for patients with herniated discs.

CHAPTER FOUR

CAREFUL MANAGEMENT

Pain Relief Techniques: Pharmaceuticals And Physiotherapy

Physical therapy and medication are frequently used in conjunction for the management of pain in herniated discs.

Pain and inflammation can be lessened with the aid of medications. NSAIDs, such as ibuprofen or naproxen, are nonsteroidal anti-inflammatory medicines that help relieve pain and reduce inflammation.

Since paracetamol lacks anti-inflammatory qualities, it can also be used to relieve pain. Stronger drugs, like opioids or muscle relaxants, may be administered in some situations, but because of their potential for dependency and adverse consequences, they are usually only used for temporary relief.

A crucial component of the conservative management of herniated discs is physical therapy.

A physical therapist can create a personalized training plan to increase flexibility, strengthen the muscles supporting the spine, and encourage good posture.

Stretches, exercises for strengthening the core, and low-impact aerobic activities like walking or swimming can all be included in this list of exercises. In addition, physical therapy sessions m

ay incorporate methods like electrical stimulation, ultrasound, heat or ice therapy, or other approaches to help reduce discomfort and accelerate healing.

Lifestyle Changes: Exercise, Weight Management, And Posture

Making lifestyle changes is essential for controlling herniated discs and avoiding new damage. Maintaining the natural curve of the spine and minimizing strain on it need good posture. This entails sitting, standing, and carrying heavy objects while keeping your spine in a neutral position. Additionally, ergonomic modifications to seating and workspace configurations can aid in improving posture and minimizing pain.

To improve general spinal health and strengthen the muscles surrounding the spine, regular exercise is essential. Walking, swimming, and cycling are examples of low-impact workouts that can assist in maintaining core strength and flexibility without placing undue strain on the spine.

But, as they might aggravate the symptoms of a herniated disc, high-impact exercises and those that require twisting or bending the spine should be avoided.

To lessen the strain on the intervertebral discs and lessen the stress on the spine, it is imperative to maintain a healthy weight. Because it puts more strain on the spine, being overweight can cause herniated discs to form or worsen.

A healthy weight can be attained and maintained with the support of a balanced diet and frequent exercise. This can reduce symptoms and enhance overall spine health.

Acupuncture And Chiropractic Care

Some people with herniated discs find that alternative treatments like chiropractic adjustments and acupuncture are helpful. Manual spine manipulation is used in chiropractic adjustments to realign vertebrae and release pressure from damaged discs. The goals of these modifications are to lessen pain, lessen nerve irritation, and enhance spinal alignment. Even while some people may experience short-term relief from chiropractic therapy, it's crucial to speak with a healthcare professional before receiving any spinal manipulations, particularly if there are questions regarding the treatment's suitability or safety.

Another complementary therapy is acupuncture, which uses tiny needles inserted into certain body locations to reduce pain and encourage healing. Acupuncture treatments have been reported to provide pain relief and better mobility in some herniated disc patients. To completely comprehend the advantages and restrictions of acupuncture for herniated discs, more study is necessary as the data for its efficacy in this situation is conflicting. Before beginning treatment, as with any alternative therapy, it's crucial to speak with a licensed professional and go over the advantages and disadvantages of the plan.

Steroid Injections Epidural

An approach for treating herniated disc pain that is less intrusive is epidural steroid injections (ESIs). A local anesthetic and corticosteroid medicine are frequently given into the area surrounding the spinal cord and nerve roots during this treatment. The anesthetic offers temporary comfort, and the steroid medicine helps to lessen inflammation and pain.

By temporarily relieving the pain and discomfort brought on by herniated discs, ESIs can improve a patient's ability to engage in physical therapy and other conservative treatments. It's crucial to remember that ESIs are a temporary fix and may need to be repeated on a regular basis to provide ongoing pain relief. Moreover, infection, nerve injury, and transient elevations in blood sugar levels in diabetics are among the possible hazards and adverse effects linked to ESIs. Thus, before moving further, it's crucial to go over the possible advantages and disadvantages of this treatment choice with a healthcare professional.

CHAPTER FIVE

SURGICAL MEDICATION ACTIONS

Surgical operations may become essential if conservative therapy is not successful in relieving the symptoms of a herniated disc. The purpose of surgery is to relieve pressure on the injured nerve and reduce any pain or discomfort that may be felt. Surgical operations exist in a variety of forms, each with unique considerations and results.

Surgical Procedure Types

Discectomy: This operation involves removing the herniated disc fragment that is pushing against the spinal cord or nerve root. Pain and other herniation-related symptoms may be lessened by relieving pressure on the nerve caused by the bulging disc material.

Microdiscectomy: A tiny incision and specialized instruments are used in this minimally invasive operation, which is similar to a regular discectomy. This method minimizes injury to surrounding tissues and allows for faster recovery times.

Fusion: Fusion surgery could be advised if the herniated disc has resulted in severe degeneration or instability in the spine. Fusion is the process of fusing two or more vertebrae together with rods, screws, and bone grafts. In doing so, the spine is stabilized and motion between the injured vertebrae is stopped.

Benefits And Risks Of Surgery

Surgical procedures for herniated discs have advantages and disadvantages, just like any medical therapy. Pain and other symptom reduction, increased mobility, and the possibility of going back to regular activities are some of the advantages. Nevertheless, there are dangers associated with surgery, including the potential for complications like persistent discomfort, bleeding, infection, and nerve injury.

Surgery Preparation: What To Expect

Patients with a herniated disc will usually be thoroughly evaluated by their healthcare professional prior to surgery. To determine the degree of the herniation and confirm the diagnosis, imaging studies like CT or MRI scans may be necessary. Additionally, patients will be given advice on how to get ready for surgery, which may involve quitting some medications and fasting the night before.

Patients usually check in at the hospital or surgical center the day before the procedure and go through preoperative procedures, such as the administration of anesthesia. Subsequently, the surgical team will carry out the selected operation, which might be a fusion, microdiscectomy, or discectomy, with the intention of reducing pressure on the damaged nerve and stabilizing the spine.

Rehabilitation And Postoperative Care

Patients will need to recuperate and rehabilitate after surgery to maximize results and reduce problems from a herniated disc. This can need a few days of observation and pain control in the hospital before being sent home. Instructions on how to manage discomfort, take care of the surgical site, and progressively get back to their regular activities will be given to patients.

Exercises for physical therapy and rehabilitation are frequently advised in order to increase flexibility and mobility and strengthen the muscles that surround the spine. Patients should pay close attention to the advice given by their healthcare professional and show up for all planned follow-up sessions in order to track their progress and resolve any issues.

Other Surgical Choices

For some herniated disc instances, additional surgical techniques may be considered in addition to standard surgical procedures such as discectomy, microdiscectomy, and fusion. These could include less intrusive methods with the potential for quicker recovery periods and less tissue damage, including endoscopic discectomy or laser spine surgery.

To choose the best course of action for their unique circumstances, patients must, however, weigh the advantages and disadvantages of these other options with their healthcare professionals.

Certain people might not be good candidates for these treatments, and results might change based on things including the location and degree of the herniation.

CHAPTER SIX

REPAY AND RESUMMATION

Early Stage Recuperation: Rest And Adjustment Of Activities

Rest is essential for the wounded area to heal in the early phases of recuperation from a herniated disc.

This is avoiding activities that exacerbate your symptoms rather than total bed rest. Here, altering one's activities is crucial. It entails modifying your everyday schedule in a straightforward way to lessen the tension on your spine.

This could entail avoiding strenuous lifting, bending over, or spending extended amounts of time sitting still without moving. Instead, concentrate on soft postures and motions that release pressure from the afflicted area.

During this phase, your healthcare professional can suggest particular stretches or exercises to help with pain relief and increased mobility. These could concentrate on the muscles that support and stabilize the spine. They might also advise applying heat or ice therapy to ease pain and minimize inflammation.

Exercises In Physical Therapy For Strengthening And Flexibility

An important part of the recovery process for a herniated disc is physical therapy. A personalized training regimen will be created by your physical therapist based on your unique requirements and skills. These exercises usually aim to increase the range of motion and flexibility while also strengthening the muscles that support the spine.

Gentle stretches to increase flexibility and lessen spinal stiffness are common workouts. In order to offer stability and support, strengthening exercises frequently concentrate on the core muscles, which include the lower back and abdominals. Every exercise will be guided by your physical therapist, who will make sure you are using the right form and technique to avoid future damage.

Pain Control Throughout Healing

An essential part of recovering from a herniated disc is pain management. To help with discomfort relief, your healthcare professional might suggest over-the-counter or prescription drugs. These could include painkillers like acetaminophen or ibuprofen and nonsteroidal anti-inflammatory medications (NSAIDs) to lessen inflammation.

Other methods of pain control could be helpful in addition to medicine. These could include of massage, acupuncture, heat or cold therapy, and chiropractic adjustments. It's critical to let your healthcare practitioner know about any changes in your symptoms and your level of discomfort so they can modify your treatment strategy.

Resuming Regular Activities: Employment, Athletics, And Leisure

It may take some time to return to your regular activities after a herniated disc injury. It's critical to pay attention to your body and raise activity levels gradually as tolerated. On whether it's safe to resume employment, sports, and other activities, your healthcare provider may offer advice.

To lessen the strain on your spine when you return to work, you might need to adjust your workplace or make some accommodations. This can entail switching up your work tasks as necessary, taking regular breaks, or utilizing ergonomic furnishings.

Similar to this, it's crucial to start out cautiously and build up your intensity over time when picking up sports or hobbies again. To avoid getting hurt again, pay attention to how your body reacts and modify as necessary.

Extended-Duration Rehabilitative Techniques

The major goals of long-term rehabilitation techniques are to protect the spine and stop further damage. To maintain the strength and flexibility of the muscles surrounding the spine, this may entail carrying on with your regular exercise regimen, which includes strength and flexibility training.

A healthy weight can help lessen the tension on the spine and lower the chance of recurrence in addition to exercise. Overall spine health can be supported by eating a balanced diet high in fruits, vegetables, lean meats, and whole grains.

In order to lessen the strain on the spine, it's also critical to maintain proper body mechanics and posture throughout regular tasks. This entails using the appropriate form when carrying large objects, sitting and standing upright, and avoiding extended periods of time spent sitting or standing without a break.

Having routine check-ups with your healthcare practitioner will help you keep track of your progress and address any problems that may come up.

You can lessen your chance of experiencing another herniated disc episode and keep your spine in good condition for many years by adhering to these long-term rehabilitation techniques.

CHAPTER SEVEN
PREVENTIVE ACTIONS

By taking proactive measures to prevent herniated capsulitis, one can preserve spinal health and avoid the discomfort and limits that this condition can cause. Keeping proper posture is an important preventive step.

Good posture guarantees that your spine is correctly positioned whether you are sitting, standing, or lifting, which lessens the strain on the discs and capsules that might cause a herniation.

Another important preventive strategy is regular exercise. Exercises like yoga, Pilates, or weight training that target the muscles that support the spine can help preserve spinal flexibility and stability while lowering the chance of injury. Herniated capsulitis can also be avoided by avoiding repetitive actions and activities that overstress the spine.

If your activities include repeated motions, be aware of your movements and take breaks to rest and stretch.

The Value Of Preserving Spinal Health

For general health and quality of life, spinal health must be maintained. Supporting the body's weight, allowing for mobility, and shielding the spinal cord and nerves are all made possible by the spine.

You can move painlessly and smoothly and carry out daily tasks with ease when your spine is in good health.

On the other hand, poor spinal health can result in a number of issues, such as herniated capsulitis.

You may lower your chance of acquiring disorders like herniated capsulitis and experience improved mobility and comfort for the duration of your life by placing a high priority on spinal health through appropriate posture, consistent exercise, and other preventive methods.

Ergonomic Advice For Preventing Injuries

For people who spend a lot of time at a desk or performing repetitive chores, ergonomics is crucial in preventing illnesses like herniated capsulitis. Having a well-configured workspace is crucial ergonomic advice. In order to encourage proper posture and lessen the strain on your spine, adjust your chair, desk, and computer monitor. In order to prevent slouching and preserve the natural curve of your lower back, use an ergonomic chair with adequate lumbar support. In order to avoid stiffness and muscular exhaustion, you should also take frequent breaks to stretch and adjust your sitting posture. To lower the risk of spinal injury when lifting large objects, utilize proper lifting techniques including bending at the knees and keeping the object close to your body.

Stretching And Exercise Programmes

A regimen for preventing herniated capsulitis must include regular exercise and stretching. Concentrate on core-strengthening exercises like planks, bridges, and crunches; a strong core helps to stabilize and support the spine. To increase flexibility and lessen back strain, use stretching exercises that focus on the muscles that surround the spine, such as the hamstrings, hip flexors, and chest muscles. Strength training and stretching can be combined in a single workout with yoga and pilates, which will improve general spinal health and lower the chance of injury.

Supplements And Diet For Healthy Spine

In order to keep the spine healthy and avoid diseases like herniated capsulitis, nutrition is essential.

A well-balanced diet high in antioxidants, vitamins, and minerals maintains the health of the spine's discs and capsules. Include foods high in calcium, such as leafy greens, dairy products, and fortified foods, to strengthen bones and lower the chance of spinal fractures caused by osteoporosis.

Fish, nuts, and seeds are rich sources of omega-3 fatty acids, which have anti-inflammatory qualities that can help lessen pain from herniated capsulitis and reduce inflammation in the spine.

Furthermore, you may want to think about supplementing with glucosamine and chondroitin, which are believed to promote joint health and lower the risk of degenerative cartilage in the spine.

Frequent Inspections And Surveillance

Consult a physician on a regular basis to monitor the health of your spine and identify any problems early on, such as herniated capsulitis.

Your healthcare practitioner can evaluate your posture, range of motion, and general spinal health during routine checks to spot any potential issues or areas to be concerned about. In order to diagnose any underlying problems and have a better look at the spine, they could suggest imaging tests like MRIs or X-rays.

By taking charge of your spinal health and scheduling routine examinations, you can take care of any problems as soon as they arise and stop them from becoming worse and more dangerous conditions like herniated capsulitis.

CHAPTER EIGHT

MANAGING METHODS AND ASSISTANCE

Although having a herniated disc might be difficult, there are coping mechanisms and resources available to assist you in properly managing your illness.

It's critical to recognize that coping involves attending to the psychological and emotional aspects of the illness in addition to the physical symptoms.

You can lessen the impact of the herniated disc on your everyday activities and enhance your quality of life by learning coping methods.

Learning more about the illness is a useful coping mechanism. You can make more informed decisions about your health if you know what causes a herniated disc, how it affects your body, and what treatment options are available. This information can also lessen worries and fears associated with the illness, making it simpler to manage its difficulties.

Pain management is a crucial component of recovering from a herniated disc. A herniated disc frequently causes chronic discomfort, which can significantly affect your day-to-day activities.

You can attempt a variety of pain treatment methods, such as prescription drugs, physical therapy, acupuncture, and methods of relaxation like deep breathing or meditation. It may take some trial and error to find the ideal combination of treatments that work for you, so it's critical to be patient and tenacious in your efforts.

Coping Strategies And Psychological Effects Of Chronic Pain

Your mental state and general well-being may suffer as a result of persistent pain brought on by a herniated disc.

When coping with chronic pain, it's common to feel frustrated, angry, depressed, or hopeless. To properly manage these emotions, it's crucial to identify them and create appropriate coping strategies.

The psychological effects of chronic pain can be managed in part by using mindfulness and relaxation practices. Being mindful, which is focusing on the here and now without passing judgment, can assist in lowering the tension and anxiety brought on by pain. Additional methods for calming down and releasing tension include gradual muscle relaxation, guided meditation, and deep breathing.

Sustaining an optimistic mindset is crucial for managing chronic pain. Although having a herniated disc might make life difficult, you can feel better about yourself and your perspective on life by concentrating on the things you can still do rather than the things you cannot. Having understanding friends and family who are supportive of your condition can also be a source of emotional support and motivation when things get tough.

Peer Networks And Support Groups

Making connections with people who are experiencing similar things can be quite helpful when managing a herniated disc. Peer networks and support groups offer a secure and compassionate space where you may talk about your experiences, get guidance and support, and gain knowledge from people who have been in your position before.

There are many different types of support groups, such as social media groups, online forums, and in-person gatherings. Select a format that you find comfortable and that enables you to communicate with people who share your experience. During difficult times, finding inspiration and hope in the experiences and accomplishments of others can be enlightening.

Interacting With Healthcare Professionals

Good communication between you and your medical professionals is crucial to the successful management of a herniated disc.

Your physicians, physical therapists, and other medical specialists are invaluable resources that may offer direction, encouragement, and options for treatment to help reduce your symptoms and enhance your quality of life.

It's critical to be open and truthful with your healthcare professionals about your symptoms, concerns, and preferred course of treatment. Maintain a record of your symptoms, any adjustments or enhancements you observe, and any queries you have for your medical staff.

Your healthcare providers can use this information to make well-informed decisions regarding your care and to modify your treatment plan as necessary.

Maintaining A Healthy Emotional And Physical State

Maintaining equilibrium between your physical and mental health is essential when dealing with a herniated disc. In addition to controlling the condition's physical symptoms, it's critical to address the emotional and psychological effects it may have on your life.

Consider including stress-relieving and mental well-being-promoting activities in your daily routine in addition to getting therapy for your physical problems.

Exercise, pastimes, quality time with loved ones, and engaging in calming activities like yoga or meditation can all fall under this category.

When it comes to managing a herniated disc, mental health needs are equally as critical as physical health needs.

Integrating Self-Care Into Daily Routine

In order to manage a herniated disc and advance general well-being, self-care is essential.

It is possible to lessen discomfort, increase mobility, and improve your quality of life by making time for your physical, emotional, and mental well-being.

It can be as easy as scheduling regular time for enjoyable and relaxing activities to incorporate self-care into your daily schedule.

This can be taking a warm bath, reading a book, walking, or engaging in mindfulness meditation. Pay attention to your body and follow your instincts, even if it means turning down obligations or activities.

Recall that taking care of yourself is not selfish; rather, it is essential to your health and well-being. You may live a more satisfying and active life and manage the difficulties of having a herniated disc if you look after yourself.

CHAPTER NINE

COMMONLY ASKED QUESTIONS OR FAQS

Can A Disc Herniation Heal By Itself?

Although it primarily depends on the severity of the condition and the body's inherent healing ability, herniated discs may heal on their own. Conservative measures including physical therapy, rest, and pain management can often aid in the disc's progressive healing process. Natural bodily mechanisms serve to relieve pressure on the injured nerves and reabsorb the disc material that has been displaced. To find the best course of action for your particular circumstance, it is imperative that you speak with a healthcare practitioner. To guarantee that the disc is repaired properly, they can monitor your progress and offer advice on suitable therapies.

How Much Time Does It Take To Recover From Surgery?

The length of time it takes to recuperate from a herniated disc surgery depends on a number of variables, such as the procedure's nature, the patient's general health, and the severity of the disc herniation. Generally speaking, recovery periods from minimally invasive procedures are shorter than those from open surgeries. Patients usually have a period of rest and rehabilitation after surgery in order to promote optimal healing of the injured area. To assist in progressively increasing strength and mobility, doctors may prescribe light exercise and physical therapy. In order to track your recovery and address any issues, it's critical that you carefully adhere to your surgeon's post-operative instructions and show up for any follow-up consultations.

Exist Any Activities I Should Stay Away From?

It's critical to stay away from activities that could aggravate symptoms or put undue strain on the spine while recovering from a herniated disc. Your healthcare physician may advise against engaging in high-impact exercises, heavy lifting, twisting, or bending at the waist, depending on the severity of the problem. These motions may put more strain on the spine and exacerbate the herniated disc, which could result in further pain and consequences. Instead, concentrate on mild workouts that strengthen and increase flexibility without overstressing the spine, such as swimming or walking. To make sure that any activities you resume are safe for your condition, always check with your healthcare practitioner before doing so.

Is It Possible To Stop Herniated Discs From Recurring?

Although it's not always feasible to stop a herniated disc from happening, there are things you can do to lower the chance of it happening again and improve the health of your spine. The risk of disc herniation can be decreased by strengthening the muscles that support the spine and maintaining a healthy weight and posture. Regular exercise can also assist. Furthermore, using safe lifting techniques—such as bending at the knees and maintaining a straight back—can help shield the spine from damage while performing daily tasks. Additionally, it's critical to pay attention to your body and refrain from overexerting yourself because doing so raises the possibility of damage. You can lessen the chance of suffering a herniated disc recurrence and safeguard your spine by implementing these techniques into your regular practice.

If Conservative Treatments Don't Work, What Should I Do?

It is imperative that you speak with your healthcare professional to discuss other treatment choices if conservative measures like rest, physical therapy, and medication aren't working to relieve your herniated disc symptoms. In certain instances, more sophisticated therapies could be required to treat neurological symptoms or chronic pain. These could involve spinal fusions or discectomy operations to remove or stabilize the herniated disc, or epidural steroid injections to lessen pain and inflammation.

Together, you and your healthcare practitioner will decide on the best course of action based on your unique needs and preferences. To guarantee that you receive the finest care possible for your herniated disc, it is imperative that you engage in open communication with your healthcare team and actively participate in the decision-making process.

www.ingramcontent.com/pod-product-compliance
Lightning Source LLC
Chambersburg PA
CBHW071839210526
45479CB00001B/201